THE MODERN MAN GUIDE

A guide to being the
ultimate gentleman –
without the boring bits

Jake Millar

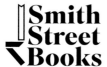

**Smith
Street
Books**

For Virg, who's the best man I know.

CON-TENTS

Don't panic. This isn't a self-help book. I'm not trying to get you to eat, pray or love yourself towards inner peace. You don't need to take up meditation during your lunch hour, or rush out to stock up on incense and a wardrobe full of clothes made from hemp. That's not what this is about.

Truth is, men used to be very different from the creatures they are today. Take fashion. Looking back even five years, many saw clothing as a practical alternative to being, say, completely naked, rather than anything to do with looking their best and expressing their personality.

These were the sort of men who thought shorts and singlets were acceptable wedding attire but – like the time they turned up to the office Christmas party sporting a Hitler moustache – those wide-eyed glances they received were not looks of admiration but pure, unbridled horror.

Cut to today. Men's fashion and grooming are now booming multi-billion dollar industries and their growth is outpacing women's equivalent markets. You probably already know this. It's the reason your social media feeds have been overflowing with men sporting perfect facial hair and suits that show a wink of ankle and jackets that actually fit. Our forefathers might have preferred to front up to a grizzly bear (or whatever men used to do) rather than face the bathroom mirror, but with anti-ageing eye serum in hand, we're now comfortable making a trip down the cosmetics aisle.

This book won't tell you what to do with your life, or demand you apply moisturiser, hairspray and a generous spritz of cologne every time you head out to the shops. After all, being the perfect gentleman is about more than just throwing on a freshly pressed pair of cream chinos. I'm pretty sure Confucius said that.

But let's get down to brass tacks – you probably came here because you need a little help. It doesn't matter if you're straight or gay, or somewhere in between; a walking Adonis or as ugly as a sack full of hammers. The next six chapters – Style, Grooming, Food & Drink, Dating, Work and Leisure – do not pretend to have all the answers for living a better life, nor will they try to turn you into some kind of poor man's Ryan Gosling, but they will give you the tools you need to be your best, most successful and stylish self.

We've a lot to cover. But by far the most important element to keep in mind is not to take all this too seriously. This is supposed to be fun. Now, let's get started.

CHAPTER ONE STYLE

Like great art or hardcore pornography, style is easy to spot but hard to define. You know it when you see it. These tips will have you standing out from the pack – for all the right reasons.

The problem with getting dressed is it sounds really simple. Short of turning up to work having neglected to put on trousers, it's hard to imagine how anything could go terribly wrong. And yet some men still manage to look like they've dressed themselves entirely in the dark, seemingly plucking items from their wardrobes at random and heading out the door. Not exactly inspiring. Instead of dressing yourself as if you've lost some kind of cruel bet, be your true, fashionable self. This chapter will give you all the tools to do just that.

WARDROBE ESSENTIALS

Think of your wardrobe like a stock portfolio. Not my stock portfolio, of course, since I'm a writer and my finances are what fancy number-crunching types might call an 'embarrassing mess'. What we're talking about is establishing a solid collection of low-risk options that will serve you well for years to come. These 10 wardrobe essentials are your blue chip stocks: the safe bets that every man needs in his closet. You can then build on them with other pieces that show more of your personality, or respond to particular fashion trends. But first, let's get the foundations in place.

A NAVY SUIT

Men just look good in suits, and that's something you'll just have to accept. A classic grey number is a strong second option – but try to avoid wearing a plain black suit to work, or you'll look like you've dropped by the office on your way to a funeral.

CHINOS

No-one wins friends with chinos. They won't be the most exciting additions to your wardrobe, but they're a handy alternative to dress trousers or jeans, and are all but impervious to style trends. Just trust me on this one.

DENIM JEANS

We're not talking about the vacuum-packed variety that make your calves look like a couple of pythons trying to digest a baby goat. Few men look good in skinny jeans – and that number decreases rapidly with age – so go for a slim, straight pair to avoid embarrassment.

WHITE SHIRTS

There's nothing better than a crisp, white shirt – except one that actually fits. Avoid anything too boxy. You want it slim in the arms and tapered at the waist – look for words like 'slim' or 'European cut' when you're out shopping.

BROGUES

Black and brown lace-ups will have you covered for most situations, from the office to an evening out. But treat them well. Keep them looking sharp by shining them regularly and resting them between wears.

T-SHIRTS

Forget your stash emblazoned with band logos or curry stains. Every guy needs a stockpile of fitted white, black and grey crew-neck (that is, round-neck) T-shirts. Wear them with jeans on the weekend, or under a suit for a stylish alternative to a formal shirt. Fun!

A BOMBER JACKET

You can't really have too many jackets. A classic black or navy zip-up bomber is great for when you want to look sharp, but when a full blazer is a little on the dressy side. Go for one that's unstructured, but slim rather than puffy.

A WINTER COAT

For warmth and breathability, pick something in wool or cashmere – or a combination of the two. If you live in a climate where even wearing long sleeves will leave you overheated, a light raincoat might be a better alternative.

SNEAKERS

Jerry Seinfeld has given the world a lot of great stuff, but his love of running shoes with jeans is not one of them. Get a fresh, white pair of low-cut sneakers (trainers). NB: these are not for doing sport.

SWEATERS

While V-neck sweaters can look like a bit worky, a crew-neck is good for all occasions. Go for black, navy or grey and you'll have plenty of options for wearing alone, or under a suit.

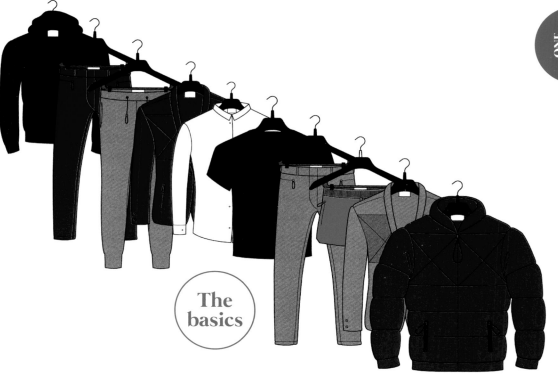

The basics

BONUS POINTS

If you've reached the age of 25, chances are you will have worn a tuxedo at least once. Renting a tux is a fool's game, because it will cost an arm and a leg, and fit like a potato sack. Not cool. A decent tuxedo will last forever and be pretty versatile, since you can wear the jacket separately with jeans and a T-shirt for a less formal look.

BLUE JEANS WERE INVENTED IN 1873 BY LEVI STRAUSS & CO. AND LATVIAN TAILOR JACOB W. DAVIS.

CLOTHING CARE

The best way to make your wardrobe last longer is to invest in good stuff to begin with. It's hardly rocket science. Buying well-made clothing, shoes and accessories pays off in the long run because even though they're likely to cost more initially, they won't need replacing often. That doesn't mean you have to apply for a second mortgage to fill your wardrobe with Italian labels, but aim for quality over quantity. Avoid too many synthetic materials, which don't last as long, tend to look worse and are often a lot less comfortable. Instead, go for natural fabrics like cotton, linen, wool or cashmere. A cheap suit might look like a good idea when you're reaching for your wallet, but your penny pinching will seem less wise when you're sitting in that important business meeting and it's cooking you like a polyester microwave. Once you've invested in some decent kit, the next step is to return the love it's shown you. Here's how to keep your clothes looking sharp.

STORING

Wire clothes hangers are not your friend. They're handy for breaking into locked cars (I hear), but they cut into fabric and will leave your clothes warped. They are also prone to rust, which can leave stains that are all but impossible to remove. Instead, kit out your wardrobe with some nice wooden hangers, which not only look much better, but are also kinder to your shirts and T-shirts. Sweaters are best folded, rather than hung, because long periods spent suspended can leave them stretched and mis-shapen. Stop your clothes from fading by storing them out of direct sunlight whenever possible, and keep suits in a dust bag for extra protection. Add some mothballs to your wardrobe to prevent insects snacking on that nice new wool jumper you bought.

WASHING

Since your parents are no longer doing your laundry (I hope?), it's time to learn the basics. Always check your garments' care directions – particularly the temperature settings – before throwing them in the machine. Delicate fabrics like silk, cashmere and some wools are best left out altogether.

Hand washing is relatively quick and painless, especially if you only have a few items. First, separate whites from colours and all-black fabrics. This is important. Then, soak all like-coloured items in a small tub of hot water for 10–15 minutes, remove and add to a separate tub filled with water and mild detergent. Submerge for around five minutes, scrub with your hands and pay special attention to any stains. Squeeze out the excess liquid and submerge in plain room-temperature water to ensure all detergent is removed. Finally, wring out any excess water and hang to dry. Some sweaters or delicate fabrics may need to be laid on a towel to 'reshape' as they dry, instead of hanging.

DRY CLEANING

Without getting too Green Peace about it all, there have long been concerns about the impact of dry cleaning solvents, in particular chlorofluorocarbons, which not only managed to get rid of stains (good), but did a great job of removing the ozone layer (bad). They've since been banned, but if you still have concerns there are more environmentally friendly alternatives to chemical dry cleaning. That said, dry cleaning has its place. If you have an office job, you'll probably be spending a lot of your time in a suit. The natural impulse is to want to take it to the dry cleaner every few days, but try to reserve this for when your suit is actually dirty – coffee spills or mishaps at lunch meetings. If the problem is just a few creases, often all it will need is a decent steam to have it looking fresh again. Buy yourself a basic hand steamer, which will sort

HOW OFTEN TO LAUNDER CLOTHING

As a general rule, err on the side of caution though if something is obviously dirty, you'll need to wash it. Don't constantly wash garments that don't really need it. Suits often require little more than airing and a quick steam, rather than a trip to the dry cleaner, which actually causes wear and tear over time. Here's a quick guide to how many times you can wear your wardrobe before you hit the laundry.

T-SHIRTS	1–2 wears
SHIRTS	1–2 wears
UNDERWEAR	1 wear (please)
SOCKS	1 wear
SWEATERS	10–15 wears
JEANS	10–15 wears
SUITS	Pretty much unlimited, providing you steam and air them regularly
COATS	Unlimited, unless visibly dirty

out any creases and will also help air out your suit after you've worn it. If you haven't got a steamer and can't be bothered getting one, a good alternative is to hang your suit in the bathroom while you take a hot shower to take care of any creases caused by everyday wear. Try to alternate which suit you wear on a daily basis and give each one a break between wears, so the creases don't become set in.

SHOE CARE

You can tell a lot about a man from his shoes, so treat them well. Use a quality leather protector, which will help guard against stains and water damage. Make sure you test the product on a small, hidden area, rather than slathering it all over your shoe. Then, invest in some shoetrees. Not only do they help your shoes keep their shape, but wooden versions also absorb moisture left by you and the elements, which can cause the leather to warp or crack. Place them into your shoes after each use, and avoid wearing the same shoes on consecutive days. If you get caught in a serious downpour, take them off as soon as you get home and stuff them with newspaper to absorb most of the water. When they're almost dry, insert a shoetree to soak up the last of the moisture and ensure the shoes stay in shape.

RECYCLING

We're not talking about separating your paper from the plastics (although best to do that, too), but about keeping a handle on your wardrobe. Unless you want to end up in an episode of *Hoarders*, you'll want to regularly update and declutter your closet. They say we wear 20 per cent of our clothes 80 per cent of the time, which means you probably have an awful lot of stuff that you never wear. The answer is to just get rid of it. Anything you haven't worn in six months should be donated or sold. Be ruthless. Are you really going to wear that Hawaiian shirt you got on vacation two years ago? Please do not.

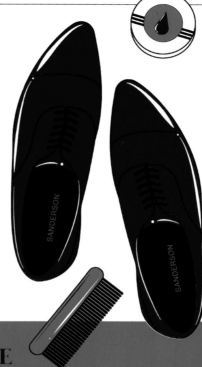

Buff up

HOW TO SHINE YOUR SHOES

Get yourself a dry cloth or chamois, shoe polish the same tone as the leather, and a shoe brush. Then, follow these steps:

1. Clean the shoes with the cloth to remove any dirt.
2. Apply a small amount of polish, using the brush.
3. Allow to dry.
4. Brush to remove any excess polish.
5. Use the cloth to buff until looking shiny and new.

TAILORING

The real issue holding many men back in the style stakes is not so much taste or budget or even a weird penchant for 'jazzy' ties. No, what's separating the men from the boys is actually pretty simple: fit. You've probably spotted them on your daily commute – men who look like they've borrowed their dads' suits, swimming along in oversized jackets and shapeless trousers that hang from their belts like curtains and have more legroom than your average Land Cruiser. The solution is tailoring. A few skilled snips and tucks can take a good suit, shirt or pair of pants and turn it into a great one.

But the battle for perfectly fitted clothes starts before you even take them home from the shop. Not all brands are created equal, and while some may go for a slimmer fit, others might cut their jacket arms especially long, or trousers particularly wide. Find labels that fit you reasonably well and where the cut suits your body shape right off the rack, so any additional nips and tucks are kept to a minimum. Good tailoring can be costly, and while having a couple of darts put in the back of your dress shirt is easy enough, getting a jacket sleeve or trouser leg slimmed down is not going to be cheap. Next time you're buying a suit, look out for the key areas on the following page.

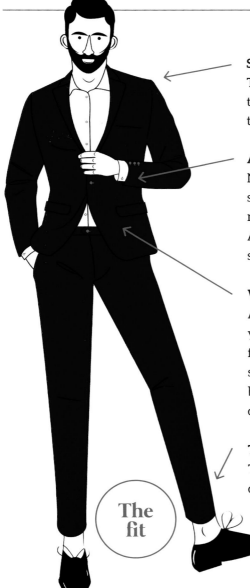

SHOULDERS

The shoulder seam should finish on the point of your shoulder, rather than slipping down your arm.

ARMS

Nothing ruins a suit like fat, billowy sleeves, so ensure they're fitted but not so tight you can't actually move. Aim for around two centimetres of shirt cuff to show at your wrist.

WAIST

Aim for fitted but comfortable, so you're able to hug someone without feeling like you're about to blow a seam. On a three-button jacket, the buttoning rule is: middle anytime; top only with middle; and bottom never.

TROUSERS

Tradition dictates one 'break' – that crease of fabric that falls around the shin, as the material rests on your shoe. But for a more modern look, feel free to show a little ankle.

The fit

ONLINE SHOPPING

For many men, clothes shopping is a task up there on the fun spectrum along-side deliberately sticking forks in your eyes or listening to your parents talk about their vigorous sex life. It usually means a couple of solid hours spent being interrogated by some hipster twenty-something about your plans for the weekend, and having to pretend you're doing something extremely fun, while knowing full well you're actually staying home to eat pizza from the box and binge on whatever you can find on Netflix. Again. Happily, that's where online shopping comes in.

Admittedly, the early years of online shopping weren't great, with lengthy and expensive delivery and tricky return policies. But you can now browse literally hundreds of items from the comfort of your own home (or bus, or train or – let's be honest – desk at work) in a way that's fast, efficient and relatively pain-free, as long as you follow a few simple rules.

KNOW YOUR MEASUREMENTS

Get a friend or tailor to take some accurate body measurements, and keep them up to date. The key areas to look out for are your waist, leg, neck and chest, as these will give a pretty good idea of how most garments will fit. Check to see what sizes you're shopping in because European, Japanese, UK and US sizing can often differ. The best option is to look at the actual measurements of the pieces you're buying and then compare them to your own.

PLAY IT SAFE

Online shopping is not really the place to throw caution to the wind. Stick with brands you know reasonably well as you will already have a pretty good idea of how their clothing will fit your body. The same goes for trying new styles, because although it might look good on the fit model, that's kind of the point – it always looks good on the fit model. Since you can't try it on, shop within your comfort zone.

READ REVIEWS

The best way to know what to expect with an online store is to read users' reviews of their experience. Pay particular attention to any delays with delivery, or nasty disputes about returning purchases, which should raise red flags. It might also be handy to read comments about particular brands to see how they fit.

DON'T FORGET THE FINE PRINT

Some websites have free returns, while others will sting you with the full cost of returning the items, which can be expensive. Try on clothing as soon as it arrives, rather than waiting and risking losing the return period. Also, know the customs requirements for your area, as you don't want to be stung when you're trying to get your stuff back into the country.

DRESS CODES

There are few experiences as embarrassing as being the only man in jeans at an event full of suits. But deciphering what to wear needn't be a case of cracking the Enigma Codes. Don't be left scratching your head every time you receive an invitation. Here are the five most common dress codes and how to nail them:

SMART CASUAL

While this is as relaxed as dress codes tend to come, the emphasis is on the smart, rather than the casual. Go for a button-up shirt, with jeans or chinos and brogues or dressy sneakers (trainers). You can probably give the tie a miss, but you might want to throw on a casual blazer or sports coat, since it's always better to be over-dressed than under. Remember that.

LOUNGE SUIT

Sometimes called 'cocktail', this is a step below a full black-tie look and tends to be more common for daytime events. While it's not set in stone, the safest bet is to wear a nice grey or navy suit – something with a pattern is good, but avoid anything black. Go for brogues or loafers, and a tie is optional. Think film stars attending the Cannes Film Festival, rather than the Oscars.

BLACK TIE

It's not quite as strict as it used to be, and these days you can swap a classic black tuxedo for a dark navy version. But other than that, stick with a white dress shirt, black tie and patent-leather shoes.

WHITE TIE

Unless your phone contacts include European royalty or Elton John, you probably won't have too many opportunities to wear white tie. A classic throwback to more formal times, this calls for a white bow tie and shirt with a black tuxedo jacket – or one with tails, if you feel like taking it up a notch.

RACE DAY

Racing carnivals are a category of their own. While most traditional race days are usually pretty dressy, different events often require very specific dress codes – some might let you show a little personality, while others might be strict black-and-white affairs. Best to check ahead of time to find out which dress code applies to the race you're attending, and pay special attention to things like whether you need to wear a jacket or tie at all times, or if a corsage is required.

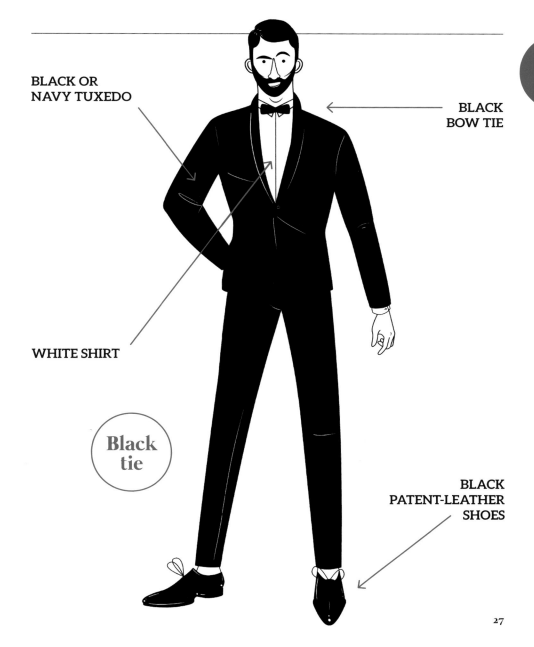

BLACK OR
NAVY TUXEDO

BLACK
BOW TIE

WHITE SHIRT

Black
tie

BLACK
PATENT-LEATHER
SHOES

CHAPTER TWO
GROOM-ING

Put your best face forward with these tips on hairstyles, fragrances and beating the clock that will have you looking your best – at any age.

There was a time when men did little more than ruggedly run a hand through their hair and walk out the door. Then the metrosexuals arrived. With their hair products and moisturisers and anti-ageing serums, too much time in front of the bathroom mirror wasn't nearly enough. Not everyone is going to spend hours getting ready each morning, but at least now we've got the tools for the job. From essential products to hairstyles, choosing the right fragrance and ageing, this chapter has all your grooming needs covered.

BATHROOM ESSENTIALS

In case you missed the memo, the days of men stealing their partners' grooming products have now faded from memory. And rightly so. Men's hair and skin have different needs than women's, and while everyone is unique when it comes to their morning routine, the basic necessities of the bathroom cabinet remain fairly standard, starting with these 10 key items:

MOISTURISER

Wrinkles, redness and blemishes show up more easily on dry skin, so moisturise every morning to give your face a healthy glow. But go for one that's matt because looking shiny is not cool.

CLEANSER

Dirt and grime, including nasties like car exhaust fumes and cigarette smoke, can start to pile up through-out the day. Use a cleanser every morning and evening to have your skin looking its best.

SUNSCREEN

The sun is not kind to your skin. Try to wear sunscreen every day (yes, really), but go for something light rather than the thick greasy stuff you wear to the beach.

A HAIR DRYER

While you don't want the cheapest model on the market, it's probably not worth shelling out for a top-of-the-line version. Get one with adjustable temperature and power settings, as well as an adapter for different kinds of styling.

COLOGNE

Every man needs at least one signature scent, though you might want to consider a couple – one for everyday use, and another for when you're going out.

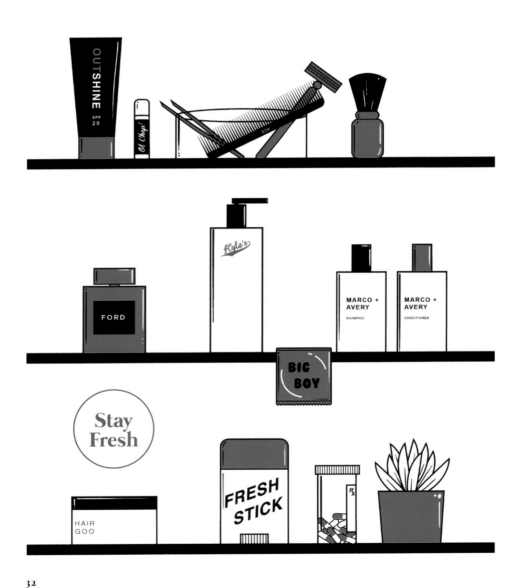

A COMB

Instead of a basic plastic model from your local supermarket, pay a little more to get a decent acetate comb that has both thick and fine teeth for versatile styling.

HAIR PRODUCT

Whether it's wax, clay or paste, find out what your hair needs and the best tool for controlling it. Ask your hairstylist to recommend something that suits your look.

SHAMPOO AND CONDITIONER

All-purpose shampoo and conditioners are fine for most types, though you might want to look out for something that moisturises, thickens or combats dandruff, depending on what your hair needs.

DEODORANT

It's pretty simple: antiperspirants fight sweat; deodorants target odour. Find out which one works for you and try to get something as natural as possible. If you wear cologne, avoid anything with a strong scent.

TWEEZERS

Keep your eyebrows from going wild with regular maintenance. Though be careful to ensure you don't end up looking lopsided.

CLEAN SHAVE

If you're going for a fuzz-free look, consider investing in a proper badger-hair shaving brush. It will help create an even lather, soften and raise your facial hair, and even help exfoliate your skin.

HAIR

When it came to men's hair product, grease – for far too long – was the word. But applying a thick coat of gel is no longer the only option, with more clays, foams, waxes and pastes on the market than you can poke a stick at. Picking the product that's right for you starts with finding your perfect hairstyle – and then tending to any other hairy areas.

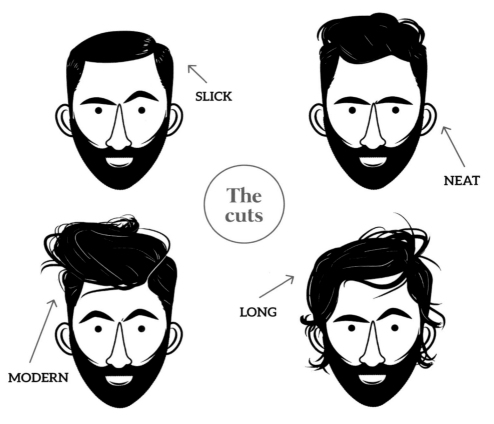

SLICK

NEAT

The cuts

MODERN

LONG

KEY HAIRSTYLES

Trust the experts. The work experience kid at your local Speedy Cuts™ might be cheap, but he's unlikely to do anything other than butcher your precious locks. Instead, find an experienced hairstylist who you get on well with (this is important) and who can suggest styles that work with your face shape, hair type and personality. Here are four key looks to consider, what to ask for in the salon, and how to recreate them at home:

Slick

What to ask for: A modern fade on the sides, and a defined part on top.
How to style it: Towel dry hair until damp and apply a small amount of pomade, which is similar to wax but gives a slicker finish. Then blow-dry while styling with your fingers. Once hair is dry, add a little more pomade with your fingertips, then use a comb to slick back. Add a little hairspray to set it in place.

Neat

What to ask for: A similar cut to slick, but with more length on the back and sides, and added texture on top.
How to style it: Don't go for anything too shiny. Apply a small amount of matt clay from the back, then style with your fingers, for a slightly less defined part.

HAIR PRODUCT

Rub a small amount onto the palms of your hands, then apply to your hair from the back, working forwards. Less is better, since you can always apply more if needed.

Modern

What to ask for: A scissor cut around the back and sides, keeping some texture and length – almost like a modern take on an undercut. Don't take much length off the top, though. How to style it: Blow-dry hair and apply a small amount of paste. Use your hands to brush into place to give it plenty of movement. Aim for rugged, not messy.

Long

What to ask for: A longer, textured cut, with plenty of volume up top. How to style it: Apply a texture spray to damp hair, then blow-dry and use your fingers to style back. Add some pomade, but go easy on the shine or you'll find yourself in Johnny Depp territory. And we're not talking the early years.

CHOOSING A HAIRSTYLIST

Getting a decent haircut starts with picking the right person for the job. The best option is to ask around and get recommendations from friends, or from online reviews. Find a place that suits your budget and your style – if you work in finance, a funky hipster salon is probably not the place to get your short back and sides. Next, go in for a consultation. A decent hairstylist will ask you not only what you want done, but also questions about your background – job, style, anything you hate – to come up with a look that will work for you. Best not to start out with anything too radical, and remember that communication is key, so keep them posted on what you're loving (or not) about your latest cut.

FACIAL HAIR

It's making a comeback in a big way. Blame the hipsters. The first step in growing some facial furniture is deciding what style and length you're going for. A full beard takes commitment, since the early stages are often not pretty. No matter how itchy it gets, resist the urge to scratch

TATTOOS

For a first-timer, best to get tattooed somewhere it can't be easily seen – away from forearms, hands or (dear God) neck and face. As much as it might seem rock and roll to get tattooed after a big night out, just don't. The chances of a drunken tattoo turning out well are slim to none. Other than that, here are a few other things to keep in mind:

- Consider what you want before you go to the tattoo parlour, instead of turning up and picking something out of a catalogue. Remember: this will be on your body forever.
- Shop around and ask some people you know who have nice tattoos for recommendations.
- Don't be thrifty. Good tattoos aren't cheap, and cheap tattoos aren't good.
- Triple-check the spelling of any words.
- Seriously consider if you want a portrait of a loved one – no-one wants to see a version of a beloved granny that looks like a reflection from one of those warped mirrors you see at the circus.
- Oh, and best not to get your current partner's name. It's just a bad idea.

'… GREY HAIR LOOKS GOOD ON EVERYBODY BUT YOURSELF.'
— KENNY ROGERS

or you can end up with problem areas or ingrown hairs. Once the hair has reached the desired length, be sure to trim it regularly to stop it getting unruly. You also want to make sure your beard or moustache is kept clean. Use a facial cleanser every morning and evening to make sure it's free of stray sandwich chunks. If you're rocking some serious length, you might even want to go for a shampoo and conditioner, as well as beard oil, which helps keep your facial hair soft, and prevents you developing dry, flaky skin. Trim your moustache when the hair is dry, since this gives you the best indication of its natural shape, and use a small amount of moustache wax to style it into place.

DOWN THERE

You need only look to the razor aisle of your local supermarket to see that this area of grooming has gone south, fast. Call them beard trimmers or body-hair razors, but let's cut to the chase: men are trimming, shaving and otherwise paying a lot more attention to their gentlemen's parts in increasing numbers. Blame porn. While there's something odd (and very itchy) about super-smooth tackle, it makes sense to trim the hedges a little bit, especially if you're particularly hirsute. Use an electric beard trimmer (not the same one you use on your face) to cut back any serious fuzz, then use a closer attachment to trim to the desired length.

If you want to shave your balls, the first priority is to take your time. Do not do it right before heading out on a date. Use plenty of shaving cream or gel, and pull the skin taut so the area you're targeting is smooth. Use slow, steady strokes with the razor and rinse regularly with hot water. Good luck.

COLOGNE

Fragrances are big business. There are literally thousands of them on the market – at least 18 courtesy of renowned tastemaker Paris Hilton – so choosing a signature scent may mean a little trial and error. You want to be sure you've made the right decision by picking something that works for you – and that you won't get sick of after a couple of days' wear.

KNOW YOUR CATEGORIES

Fragrances are generally divided into three main groups: citrus, green and spicy. Citrus tends to be fresh and summery like lemon or tangerine; green fragrances have notes like fig or star anise; and spicy scents are usually richer and leathery. Narrow down your search by reading reviews of fragrances to determine the category they fit in, and try them to find which of the three types work best for you.

TAKE A FRIEND

Having someone with you is about more than moral support. They'll be able to give you an honest opinion on what they think works – and what doesn't. Often if you're trying a lot of different fragrances in one go, the scents can become overwhelming, so it pays to have someone there who can lend a fresh nose.

BE PATIENT

Most scents have three layers: top, middle and base notes, and each develops over time. The top note usually appears after a few seconds, but the middle and base notes can take a couple of hours to fully develop. While you might not be able to stand around in a department store for several hours – well, not without a few odd looks, anyway – it pays to wait as long as you can to allow the fragrance to fully develop on your skin. Sometimes fragrances can seem mild at first, but can build to a heavier scent you're no longer keen on.

SHOP AROUND

Good fragrances aren't cheap. But rather than going for something budget, invest in a decent one that will smell better and last longer on your skin. It often pays to shop online, but there are a lot of fakes out there – make sure you're browsing reputable sites before you buy.

HOW TO
APPLY COLOGNE

We've all known someone whose fragrance arrives like a punch in the face. Don't be that guy. Spraying a fragrance directly onto yourself after you've dressed is a recipe for overdosing – and might even stain your clothing. Aim for areas that come into contact with the air most often – the neck and wrists – and if you're still unsure whether you've gone overboard, ask a friend to give you an honest opinion. These steps will ensure you apply the right amount, every time:

1. Shower and dry skin.
2. Deliver one spray to each wrist.
3. Dab each side of your neck, or spray directly into the air above and allow to 'mist' over you.
4. Allow to dry before getting dressed.

THE GLOBAL
FRAGRANCE
INDUSTRY IS
ESTIMATED TO
BE WORTH OVER
AU$50 BILLION
A YEAR.

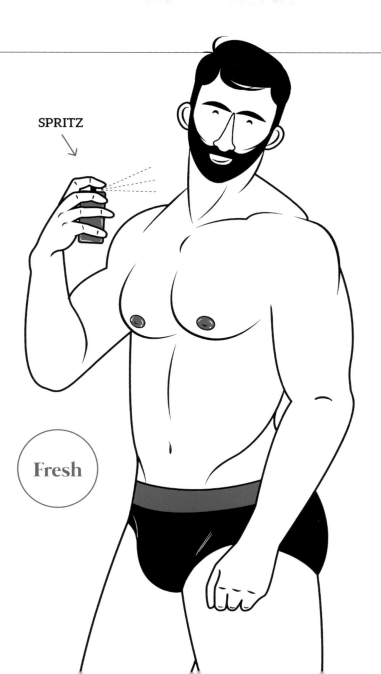

SPRITZ

Fresh

> ## WHERE TO STORE COLOGNE
> Some suggest refrigerating fragrances makes them last longer. But if you're not planning to keep them for years, a cool, dry place, out of direct sunlight is usually fine.

AGEING

Time can be a cruel mistress. None of us are getting any younger, but rather than growing depressed about the gradual march of the years, you might as well handle it with dignity. Few sights are as sad as a man desperately clinging onto his youth. But resigning yourself to the effects of age doesn't mean giving up on life, letting your hair grow out and binging on pizza all day. It's about embracing the fact that your latter years have just as much to give you as your more youthful ones – including wrinkles.

FACE

The boring reality about anti-ageing is that the best defence against the effects of time is also the most obvious: prevention. No-one who's spent a lifetime tanning at the beach or sucking down cigarettes by the packet wants to hear that, but it's the truth.

When it comes to your skin, the sun is one of the worst offenders. Ignore this, and you'll look like a leather handbag by the time you hit middle age. Go for a sunscreen that's at least SPF 30+ and apply it to your face every day, even when it is overcast. Use a facial cleanser twice a day, and a moisturiser every morning to conceal any fine lines or blemishes. You may want to also use an anti-ageing cream – particularly in problem spots under the eyes – to tighten your skin and slow the signs of ageing.

HAIR

Losing your hair is a real kick in the balls. But the problem is not so much that men lose their hair, but the importance society places on it. If we took half the money we blow on tackling baldness and spent it on medical research, cancer would probably be an issue of the past. Still, if your hairline is retreating as time advances, the worst decision you can make is to fight it – think bad comb-overs; toupees; whatever Donald Trump has done to his head. None of those are the right answer. Embrace your hair loss and shave or trim what's left, rather than clinging onto the last few strands. Trust me: it looks better than you think. As for hair colour, think long and hard before you start dyeing. If you're grey long before your time, it makes sense to delay the inevitable, but most of the time it looks obvious on more senior gents. Plus, if you start in middle age, when do you stop? Jagger's still getting about on stage with lush, brunette locks, but he's only kidding himself. There's nothing wrong with letting nature take its course. It's worked out OK for George Clooney.

INTERVENTION

While women often get a lot of flack for what they do to their faces, men are increasingly joining the anti-ageing party by getting injections, peels and lifts to fight back the years. But it's a slippery slope, and we've all seen men who've gone off the deep end – their foreheads buffed to the texture of a bowling ball; eyebrows hoisted north in that expression of the very rich or very surprised. It's fine if you want to go down that path but be wary that once you start it's very hard to stop. Here's looking at you, Kenny Rogers.

CHAPTER THREE
FOOD & DRINK

Few sights are as impressive as a man who's confident in the kitchen. Whether it's knife skills or preparing the perfect martini you're after, you've come to the right place.

Everyone wants to be a chef these days. But despite the sheer number of reality TV shows devoted to the pursuit, most have essentially become Big Brother with frying pans – the actual cooking having long since gone on the back burner. And in any case, when you consider that the reality of getting into the food business means years of chopping onions while being screamed at by crinkly faced Gordon Ramsay types, it really starts to lose its glamorous appeal. But just because you're not about to land a Michelin star, doesn't mean you should use your oven for nothing more than storage.

KITCHEN BASICS

Believe it or not, culinary essentials extend beyond operating a barbecue scraper and sporting one of those aprons with big plastic boobs. Even if you're not about to invest in some chefs' whites anytime soon, it's worth learning how to do the basics.

How to ...

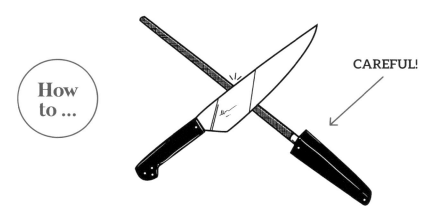

CAREFUL!

SHARPEN A KNIFE

- Take your sharpening steel with your non-dominant hand, and hold vertically, with the tip against a chopping board.
- Hold your knife against the rod, at around a 15–20 degree angle.
- Starting with the base of the knife, run it downwards towards the chopping board.
- Gradually pull the knife back, so the tip of the blade is in contact with the steel.
- Do this three to six times, depending on how dull your knife is.
- Flip the knife in your hand, so the blade is now facing upwards and repeat the process.

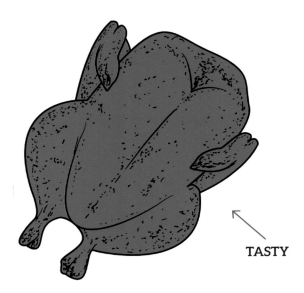

TASTY

BREAK UP A CHICKEN

- With the chicken breast-side up, pull each leg away from the body, then slice through between the breast and the drumstick.
- Pull the leg away from the body, exposing the joint, and cut through the joint and skin until completely removed.
- With the legs removed, place the chicken on its side and repeat the process with the wings.
- Place the chicken with the breast-side up, lift the breast slightly and cut downward through the rib cage to separate.
- Turn the chicken breast-side down and cut through the centre bone.
- Take each chicken breast and cut through the bone horizontally.
- With a bit of luck, you'll end up with eight pieces.

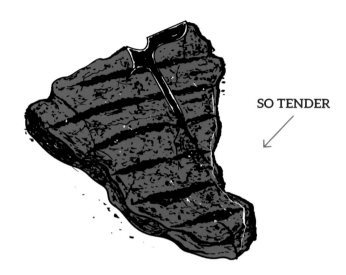

SO TENDER

THREE

COOK A STEAK

- Buy decent meat. Nothing good comes of cheap steak.
- Take it out of the fridge and allow to reach room temperature.
- Rub each side with a little olive oil and plenty of salt and pepper.
- Take a grill pan and heat until very hot. If the steak is especially thick, turn it down slightly so as not to burn the outside while the inside remains raw.

- For a 3.5 cm (1½ in) fillet steak:
  Rare (seared but still red in the centre): about 2.5 minutes each side.
  Medium rare (half seared on outside, half red inside): around 3.5 minutes each side.
  Medium (seared on outside, with thin channel of pink inside): 4 minutes each side. Any longer, and you're eating leather.
- Rest for 10–15 minutes.

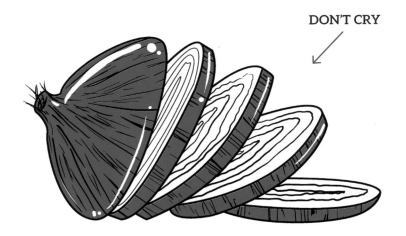

DON'T CRY

DICE AN ONION

- Cut the onion in half, from root to tip.
- Remove and discard a small amount of the root and tip, but keep the root intact, so the onion holds together.
- Peel off the outer skin, and place flat-side down on a chopping board.

- Make a series of vertical cuts, towards the root, making sure not to cut all the way through, so the onion doesn't break apart.
- Turn the onion 90 degrees and make a series of horizontal cuts the same width, from tip to root.
- Discard the remaining root.

DINNER PARTIES

At best, dinner parties are a great opportunity to avoid overzealous restaurant staff, enjoy some good old-fashioned home cooking and gossip about other people who aren't invited. What fun. At worst, they're the kind of torture that's surely forbidden by the Geneva Convention. Still, don't let that put you off. To give you and your guests the best chance of enjoying your next one, follow these few simple tips.

THE MENU

People often try to go to town with their dinner party menu, but it's about the experience – not just the food. If you're trying to impress people with your cooking, you're likely to just create extra stress. Remember to actually spend time with your guests, instead of running back and forth from the kitchen. Try to choose dishes you can prepare ahead of time – soups or slow-cooked roasts – that pretty much take care of themselves. A cheese board is a good way to finish, instead of jumping up to prepare something fancy. Plan a nice balance of light and heavy dishes, so people feel full without leaving the table groaning.

THE GUESTS

Don't go crazy. Inviting too many people rarely ends well, so go for a number you're confident cooking for. Give them plenty of notice and ask them about any food allergies or preferences. That goes for drinks, too – though it's a good idea to get people to bring anything they feel like drinking, so there's one less task to worry about. Also, don't feel you have to invite anyone you don't want to spend time with. It's your house, your rules.

THE PLAN

Make sure you have enough time to get ready before the guests arrive. Have a drink waiting for them, and choose a playlist that will last at least as long as you're planning to have them over. Have coffee or tea at the end, if you want to give people the sign it's time to go – especially if they've been stuck into the wine. Try to keep conversation polite, depending on who's attending. Steer it away from the fact that Debbie's husband's been playing around behind her back, again. No-one likes tears. It also pays to set aside some room in the fridge in case of any leftovers – though hopefully there won't be too many.

CHOOSING A DRINK

If you want to know your way around a drinks menu – or impress a date with your wine knowledge – here are a few pointers to keep in mind when you're choosing wine, beer or whisky.

WINE

There are better ways to choose a good wine than picking the second-cheapest bottle on the menu. As a general rule, wine pairing follows the same basic rules of food combinations – acidity goes well with fatty or sweet foods, in the same way you might serve a lemon wedge with avocado. Simple. Next time you're faced with the wine list, don't panic – here is a guide to matching wines with food.

Sparkling
Order: Champagne, Prosecco
Eat: Leafy green vegetables, soft or hard cheese, pasta or bread, fish

Light Dry White
Order: Sauvignon Blanc, Pinot Grigio
Eat: Leafy green or roasted vegetables, pasta or bread, fish

Sweet White
Order: Riesling, Moscato

THREE BOTTLES OF CHÂTEAU LAFITE ROTHSCHILD 1869 WERE SOLD FOR US$232,692 A BOTTLE AT AUCTION IN 2010, WHICH IS THE MOST EVER PAID FOR A BOTTLE OF WINE.

Eat: Soft cheese, pasta, cured meats, dessert

Rich White
Order: Chardonnay, Viognier
Eat: Roasted vegetables, pasta or bread, seafood, chicken

Light Red
Order: Pinot Noir, Grenache
Eat: Roasted vegetables, pasta or bread, seafood, chicken

Medium Red
Order: Sangiovese, Merlot, Tempranillo
Eat: Hard cheese, pasta or bread, chicken, red or cured meat

Bold Red
Order: Cabernet Sauvignon, Shiraz, Zinfandel
Eat: Hard cheese, red or cured meat

BEER
At its most basic, beer contains just four key ingredients: malt, hops, water and yeast. Malt typically means malted barley (barley grains that have been left in water until they begin to sprout) but alternatives include wheat or corn. Other than that, beers can generally be divided into ales and lagers, with the main difference being the yeast used in the fermentation process.

Ales
These are fermented warm, and are often stronger and fruitier than lagers – they're usually served at 'cellar' temperature, or around 10–12°C (50–55°F). Some key ales include pale ale, barley wine, stout and Belgian lambic beer.

Lagers
Typically made from cold-fermenting yeast, these are crisper, mellower and lower in alcohol – they're almost always served cold. Some lagers include pilsner, American lager, and German beers, bock or dunkel.

Key Words

Body: The sensation of the beer on your palate, from watery (light) to creamy (full).

Colour: All beers are graded from straw to black, on a scale measured by the Standard Reference Method. Low numbers describe lighter beers (wheat ales, pilsner), and high numbers refer to darker ones (stout).

Crisp: This is how carbonated or effervescent the beer is.

Hoppy: Bitter flavours are derived from the hops that balance the malt's sweetness. Fruity or citrus flavours can also be produced, depending on the hops used. 'Hoppy' flavours are most often seen in lighter beers like pilsner or pale ale.

Malty: This is a sweeter taste that comes from the malted grains used in the brewing, though they can also give a beer a darker or heavier flavour, like caramel. Darker beers like dunkel or stout tend to be malty.

WHISKY

Whole books have been devoted to the craft of whisky making and what sets each variety apart. But who's got the time? Here's a quick guide to the key things you need to know.

Process

Wondering how whisky ends up in your drink?

Grains: The most common grains used in whisky production are barley, rye, wheat and corn. Malted barley is more common in Scottish single malts, while American whiskies use more rye and corn. The grains are malted, then dried and heated.

Mashing: The cooked grains are ground into a fine flour and mixed with warm water to create a liquid called the 'mash'.

Fermentation: The mash is mixed with yeast to convert the sugars into alcohol (similar to how beer is made). This is called the 'wash'.

Distilling: The wash is heated to create alcohol vapour. The vapour is collected in a tank, and then condensed.

Ageing: Water is added and then it is stored in wooden barrels to age and develop the whisky's particular flavours.

Bottling: After the ageing process is complete, the finished product is bottled.

Varieties

Whiskies are distinguished by the grain used, their origin and the length or style of barrel ageing. Here are four key types you can expect to see:

Bourbon: US regulations require it to be made from 51 per cent corn, aged in charred white oak barrels (usually for around four years), and be at least 40 per cent alcohol per volume. It's known for its sweet caramel flavours and reddish colour.

Rye: This is made with at least 51 per cent rye mash and aged in charred oak barrels for at least two years. Rye gives the whisky fruitier notes that usually make it less sweet than bourbon.

Scotch: Single malt Scotches are made in Scotland from barley and water, and must be aged in oak barrels for at least three years. Each region lends particular characteristics to the Scotch – from the highlands, where it tends to be smokier, to the lowlands, which gives it lighter flavours.

Blended whiskies: These are generally the result of mixing a premium whisky with a less expensive one.

'I NEVER GO
JOGGING. IT
MAKES ME SPILL
MY MARTINI.'
— GEORGE BURNS

CLASSIC COCKTAILS

The rattle of ice in a shaker, that smooth tinkle of hard liquor on frosted glass: yes, it must be cocktail hour. Hooray! Yet ordering a fancy drink at a bar is often a fraught exercise. You ask the bartender – sorry, mixologist – to make you one of their finest concoctions, only to witness an elaborate series of emulsions and infusions that costs you half an hour of your life and the price of a steak dinner. Not fun. So we're harking back to simpler, better times, with five classic cocktails every man needs in his repertoire, just in case you need to entertain unexpected guests. Or yourself.

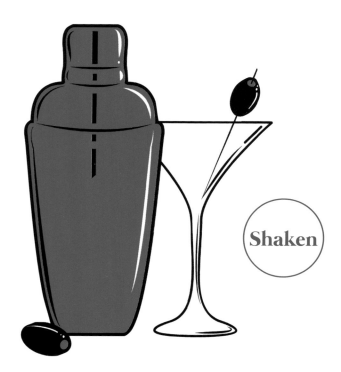

Shaken

DRY MARTINI

Use either vodka or gin, depending on your taste, and live out your Bond fantasies – minus the gunfights and womanising (probably).

INGREDIENTS
- 15 ml (½ fl oz) vermouth
- 90 ml (3 fl oz) gin or vodka
- 1 olive or lemon twist, to garnish

METHOD
- Fill a shaker with ice.
- Pour in the vermouth, and the gin or vodka.
- Quickly stir or shake for around 10 seconds, as desired.
- Strain into a chilled cocktail glass and garnish with the olive or lemon twist.

TIP
Add more vermouth for a 'wetter' martini, or less for a 'drier' one. Mix in a splash of olive brine when serving to turn it into a Dirty Martini.

THREE

OLD FASHIONED

While some trends are best confined to the 1960s – casual drink driving, chain smoking all of the cigarettes in the world – the decade gave us some pretty phenomenal drinks. This is one of them.

INGREDIENTS

- 1 sugar cube
- Angostura bitters
- soda water
- 60 ml (2 fl oz) rye whisky
- 1 orange slice or maraschino cherry, to garnish

METHOD

- Place the sugar cube in an Old Fashioned glass and wet with two or three dashes of bitters and a dash of soda water.
- Crush the sugar cube with a spoon and rotate the glass to line it with the syrup.
- Add one large ice cube and pour in the whisky.
- Garnish with an orange slice or maraschino cherry.

TIP

If you're not a big fan of brown spirits, swap the whisky for the same amount of gin.

BLOODY MARY

The ideal spicy, peppery liquid pick-me-up after a long night out, it's basically the original power juice.

INGREDIENTS
- 30 ml (1 fl oz) vodka
- 60 ml (2 fl oz) tomato juice
- worcestershire sauce, Tobasco sauce, sugar, black pepper and lemon juice, to taste
- 1 celery stick and lemon slice, to serve

METHOD
- Fill a tall glass three-quarters with ice.
- Add the vodka and tomato juice.
- Top with worcestershire and Tabasco sauce, sugar, pepper and lemon juice, as desired.
- Stir, and serve with the celery stick and lemon slice.

TIP
To make a large batch for parties (or personal use), just keep the ratio one part lemon juice to three parts vodka and six parts tomato juice.

THREE

MARGARITA

Few cocktails are butchered quite as severely as the Margarita. Stick to this classic recipe for the best, most authentic results.

INGREDIENTS

- 1 lime wedge
- 45 ml (1½ fl oz) tequila
- 30 ml (1 fl oz) Cointreau
- 45 ml (1½ fl oz) lime juice
- sea salt

METHOD

- Take a chilled cocktail glass, run the lime wedge around the rim and dip it in salt. Reserve the lime wedge.
- Fill a cocktail shaker two-thirds with ice and add the other ingredients.
- Strain into a glass and serve with the reserved lime wedge.

TIP

To make a frozen margarita (trashier, sure, but delicious), measure a cocktail shaker of ice into a blender and blitz until crushed. Add the other ingredients, blitz again quickly, then pour into a salt-rimmed cocktail glass and serve.

NEGRONI

Campari tends to split opinion. Some bemoan it as the devil's own drink, while others simply can't get enough. If you're one of the latter, this is an essential recipe.

INGREDIENTS
- 30 ml (1 fl oz) gin
- 30 ml (1 fl oz) sweet vermouth
- 30 ml (1 fl oz) Campari
- orange peel, to garnish

METHOD
- In a cocktail shaker, shake all the ingredients with ice and strain into a chilled glass.
- Garnish with the orange peel.

TIP
For a more refreshing (read, less alcoholic) alternative, take a tall glass and add plenty of ice. Pour in one part Campari to two parts soda water, and top with an orange slice.

THREE

THE MORNING AFTER

We've all been there – waking up the day after a few too many drinks and feeling like the room is spinning and your face is about to peel off. But while plenty of companies claim to have the ultimate cure – from pills and potions to intravenous injections – truth is, you probably just have to wait it out. You don't want to hear it, but prevention is the best way to stop a hangover – try not to mix drinks during the night, avoid too many sugary cocktails, and alternate alcohol with water whenever possible. Still, despite the best of intentions, we've all managed to get a bit excited from time to time.

STAY HYDRATED

Alcohol dehydrates your body, which is one of the reasons it feels like you have a vice attached to your skull right now. Drink plenty of water, especially if you're planning on having a few coffees. While some people swear by sports drinks to replace lost electrolytes, truth is there's actually not much evidence they help. Their primary benefit is to give you an energy boost, since they're often full of sugar. As for the hair of the dog, getting back on the horse and having more booze might make you feel better, but it's really just delaying the inevitable.

EAT SOMETHING

While your first instinct might be to stay in bed and then eat all the pizza in the world, the allure of greasy food the morning after is more of a craving than hard science. Eating carbohydrates can help replace some of the energy lost by your body processing alcohol, but in an ideal world, it's best to have a healthy meal and then get some rest. If you're taking painkillers, just be careful not to go overboard, as your liver is already busy processing the drinks you downed last night, and could probably do without the extra work.

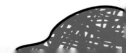

EXERCISE

Being active is the best way to cure a hangover, despite your body telling you to stay under the covers all day. Provided you've consumed plenty of water, going out for a gentle run helps your body metabolise alcohol more quickly, and will release endorphins, which make you feel better. But there is some good news – sex is another proven hangover cure, so feel free to get busy. You're welcome.

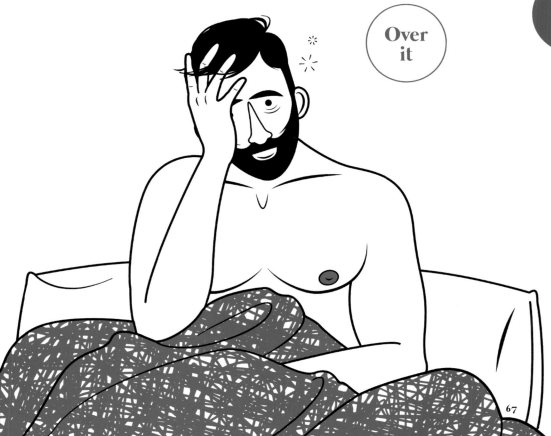

CHAPTER FOUR
DATING

Find your perfect match with these tools that will take you from successfully navigating the dating world to coupled bliss.

Don't worry if you haven't found The One because there are plenty of fish in the sea. Blah, blah, blah – you've heard it all before. There are options beyond simply resigning yourself to a lifetime of soup for one, and waiting for the cats to start adding up. From first dates, to online dating, popping the question and more, these tips will help get you on the right track to eternal love, whether you're straight, gay, or somewhere in between. Because, let's face it, we could all use a little help. Or a lot.

FIRST DATES

Meeting someone for the first time doesn't have to feel like fronting the Spanish Inquisition. Think of it as just another chance to get to know someone, and don't take it personally if it doesn't work out. After all, it's better to choose someone who's right for you than settle for a partner you don't get on well with. Good. Now we've got that sorted, here's how to make the most of it.

CHOOSE THE RIGHT VENUE

Provided you're the one choosing where to meet, try to pick somewhere you're familiar with, so there are fewer surprises and you'll already know how to get there. Best to aim for a venue about halfway between you and your date. While many immediately think of dinner for a first date, a drink might be a better option. It's a less formal way to meet some-one, and if it really goes south, it's a lot easier to make your excuses after one drink and part ways, rather than finding out you have nothing in common one plate into a seven-course degustation. Also, for safety's sake, never go to someone's house on a first date, and try to choose somewhere

relatively public. There are a lot of crazies out there.

ARRIVE ON TIME

Non-negotiable. In fact, try to arrive with plenty of room to spare – you can always pop into the bathroom for a final hair or teeth check, and get settled before they arrive. There's nothing that will throw you off your game more than running late and looking flustered. It also allows you to get acquainted with the menu, which can be a good way to break the ice. In terms of dress, you want to look smart but not too formal – a blazer and jeans is a strong option. A good alternative is to meet straight after work (we're talking business attire – not painter's

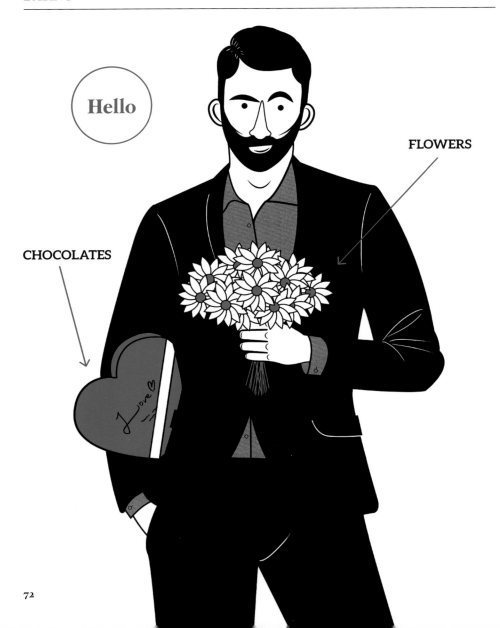

overalls), which takes any dress code worries out of the equation.

WATCH YOUR MANNERS

Not only are you meant to be on your best behaviour while you're on a date, but your partner will assume that's the case – so if you are sloppy, they'll think that's as good as you're going to get. Nothing is a bigger turn-off than someone who's rude to waitstaff, so be polite and courteous to everyone, and fill your date's glass with water or wine before yours. But take it easy on the booze or they might end up thinking you're a train wreck. Generally, whoever asked the other person on the date is obliged to foot the bill, but it never hurts to offer. If they turn you down, or ask to split it, that's fine. Don't make a huge deal of it, because no-one wants to end a date with an embarrassing arm wrestle over the cheque. You can always offer to go for a cocktail somewhere else and say you'll let them pay for it.

... AND YOUR MOUTH

Topics to avoid include the usual suspects: politics, religion, sex, your exes and sex with your exes. Also, avoid talking about work, if you can help it. While it's bound to come up, you don't want conversation to focus on the minutiae of your day because, chances are, it's not that interesting. No-one wants to go on date with someone who only talks about themselves, so try to steer conversation towards the other person. Prepare a list of interests you both share, and be prepared to talk about them. Nothing kills a first date quite like the sound of crickets.

Don't take it personally if the date doesn't work out because there are countless qualities someone might be looking for in a prospective partner, and chances are, you're not going to meet all of them. It's just simple maths. Instead, tell yourself that unlike a job interview, this is just a chance to get to know someone and if you hit it off, that's great. If not, move on.

FOUR

ONLINE DATING

There was a time when having an online dating profile guaranteed that you had a pristine collection of Star Trek figurines and parents for housemates. But with the rise of dating apps, now everyone's got an online presence. So it only makes sense to put yourself out there. As long as you follow a few simple rules, you'll have a winning profile in no time at all.

BE HONEST

Lying about your height or age might seem like a good way to attract some extra interest, but the aim here is to get people to like the real you – not someone you wish you were. When are you going to tell them you're not the head of a Fortune 500 company, or that you don't really like cats? That you actually hate cats? Not exactly a recipe for true love. After all, the best relationships are built on honesty. Be sure to include as much information about yourself as you can, including what you like to do in your spare time, your interests, your favourite movies, as well as anything that's a real deal breaker – smoking, drinking, age range and so on.

YOUR PHOTO

Make sure your face is clearly visible, but not too close. Selfies are generally a bad idea. Posting a photo of you doing something you enjoy – hiking, attending a party where you weren't wasted – is a good idea so they get to see what you look like, and you can show them one of your hobbies. Best not to include anyone else in the frame or people might wonder if that really is a friend's arm draped around you, or if you've just conveniently cropped out your partner (or spouse). Shirtless images are out if you're after a serious relationship, since it just tells people you're after a hook up. Finally, make sure your photo is recent. Nothing makes for an awkward rendezvous like a date failing to recognise you because you have half the hair they expected.

BE CAREFUL

If something seems too good to be true, it probably is. You can be gullible when you're not thinking clearly, so ask a friend's opinion if you spot something suspicious. It's easy to steal someone else's photos, so keep in mind that a busty woman unexpectedly proclaiming her love could be fibbing. And she might not even be a Nigerian princess, for that matter.

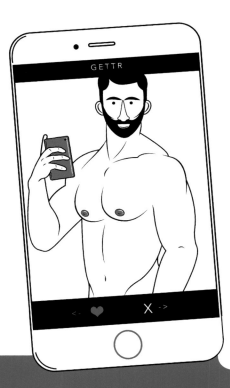

SEXTING

Breaking news: no-one wants to see a photo of your junk. Not only is it unlikely to look as impressive as you think (especially squashed into the dimensions of a phone screen), but it could also end up on the internet for all to see – even your parents. If you really can't resist the urge to send people photographs of your gear, make sure your face – or an identifying feature like a tattoo – isn't in the shot.

GETTING SERIOUS

You've been with your partner for long enough to know they're The One – and now you want to make it official. Popping the question doesn't have to be stressful, provided you know what to do and prepare ahead of time. These tips will have you covered from picking the right ring to what to say when you go down on bended knee.

CHOOSE A RING

Work out a budget and decide what you can afford. While many people think bigger is better, that's not always the case, since the clarity, cut and colour of the stone affect the way a diamond looks – and how much it'll cost. These categories are often called the 'Four Cs'. Allow me to explain.

Cut

Straight out of the ground, diamonds are not much to look at. The art of diamond cutting is what gives them the nice, shiny brilliance we know and love. There are many different 'cuts' of diamond on the market – princess, round, pear, etc. – each with their own pros and cons. Your best bet is to (subtly) find out which cut your partner prefers, and take it from there.

Carat

This is how much the diamond weighs. One carat equals 200 mg ($7/1000$ oz), and while bigger diamonds tend to cost more, it's worth noting the price tends to jump around milestone weights. For instance, a diamond that weighs exactly 1.0 carats is likely to set you back a lot more than one that's 0.99 carats.

Clarity

This is a measure of how many imperfections a stone has – faults like small cracks or whether it appears clear or cloudy. Diamonds are

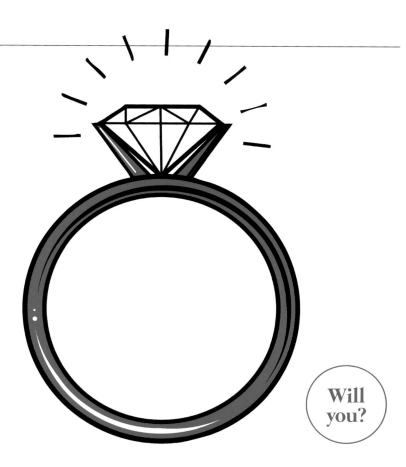

Will
you?

generally measured on a scale from imperfect (cheaper) to flawless (pricey).

Colour
Generally speaking, the clearer the diamond, the more it will cost. Stones with some degree of discolouration are considered to be less 'pure', though certain shades of diamond – pink or yellow, in particular – are extremely rare and are actually much more expensive.

WHAT TO SAY

Rather than simply dropping to one knee and asking if they'll marry you, it's best to prepare a few words about why they mean so much to you. It could be something about you knowing they were the 'one' the moment you met, or that you'd never seen anyone so beautiful. You're going for tears. Practise in front of the mirror so you don't stumble over your words, and be sure to finish with the line 'will you marry me?' so there's no confusion.

WHERE TO SAY IT

If they're chronically shy and hate football, it's probably not such a fantastic idea to pop the question on the big screen at a stadium. While a crowded fancy restaurant might seem romantic, your partner might find it a bit embarrassing to cause a scene. Try to go for somewhere that holds a certain significance in your relationship – the place you went on your first date, or a picnic in a park that has their favourite view of the city.

... AND WHEN

Weddings are not cheap. While it might not seem romantic to think of money when you're all loved up, you want to be realistic about whether you're actually in a financial position to tie the knot. If your partner has been dropping hints about marriage, that's probably a good sign. But if the relationship's quite new, and they've mentioned not being ready for marriage, it might be worth waiting it out to avoid being disappointed.

AFTERWARDS

You're not out of the woods just yet. Now they've said yes (hopefully), it's time to start telling relatives and discussing plans for when you'll walk down the aisle. But there's no rush – the average length of engagement is over a year. After all, it's better to have enough time to organise your wedding day just the way you want it than to end up with a half-baked ceremony you'll remember for all the wrong reasons.

AMERICAN GRANDMOTHER LINDA WOLFE HAS BEEN MARRIED 23 TIMES, WHICH IS MORE THAN ANYONE ELSE IN HISTORY.

BREAKING UP

If breaking up were easy, pop music would never have existed. And a world without Adele is, frankly, not one I want to live in. Getting dumped is never going to be fun, but sometimes it's best for both sides of the equation. There's nothing worse than letting a doomed relationship limp on for years, while trying to fix it by getting married or having half a dozen kids. So if it is time to call it off, here are a few pointers to do it the right way.

JUST DO IT

Use the bandaid approach and avoid putting it off. Pick somewhere private – your living room, rather than, say, a friend's dinner party – and explain why you think it's best to end the relationship. Be honest but try not to be negative. Blaming them for the end of the relationship is just going to add insult to injury, but be sure to actually say something like, 'I think we should break up' so there's no confusion about the issue.

STAY CLASSY

The key to remember is that it should be done in person, unless you want to out yourself as a complete prick.

Any other form of communication – text message, email, Post-It note – is not just a bad look, but is all but guaranteed to eventually turn you into dinner party fodder, when the topic of terrible boyfriends emerges. Doing it in person will allow you both to talk about the issue freely, and will bring closure to the situation.

BE UNDERSTANDING

They'll probably be emotional. They might be angry. They may even start hurling insults. But just accept the fact they're probably going to say a few mean things about you, and don't respond. Break-ups are difficult, and fighting back with all the reasons you're leaving them is just going to make matters worse. Also, don't make the break-up about them – though instead of the old 'it's-not-you-it's-me' line, go with be something like 'this really isn't working for me'. If you make it about something they've done wrong, they'll probably just tell you they can change.

MAKE A CLEAN BREAK

There are two kinds of people in the world: there are those who stay friends with their exes and there are those who don't. Decide which camp you fall into and stick with it. If you're not going to see them again, delete their number and don't try to contact them – especially after a few too many beers – because hooking up with your ex is almost always a bad idea. It's time to move on.

OH NO!

You've run into your ex. Seeing someone you used to date can be awkward, but it's probably going to happen from time to time. Ignoring them completely is poor form (as is diving behind a parked car), so unless things ended really badly, a simple greeting is polite. If they stop for some small talk, avoid mentioning any current partners and stick to safe topics: what they've been up to lately, how their family is, etc. Don't get mean. Don't make a scene – no matter how tempting it is to settle old scores. If you still have unresolved issues, it might be worth arranging a proper catch-up to sort things out. Nothing good comes of holding a grudge.

CHAPTER
FIVE
WORK

Excluding any surprise lottery winnings or a juicy inheritance from that great-aunt you never liked in the first place, you're going to spend a fair chunk of your life earning a living. Here's how to land your dream job, get a pay rise and survive the world of office politics.

By the time you eventually pop your clogs, you'll have spent around 20 per cent of your waking hours at work. And that's assuming you're not a workaholic (which you probably are). But rather than getting all depressed about the daily grind, you might as well make the most of it. Sit quietly in the background and you'll rarely get picked out for a promotion, forever left to wonder what might have been. Instead, with a little ambition and these few handy tips, you'll find yourself in the corner office in no time. Well, maybe.

WRITING A JOB APPLICATION

Before you have to worry about turning up to the office on time, or remembering what your boss's coffee order is, you need to actually get a job. That starts with a strong application that highlights your key strengths, skilfully glosses over your weaknesses, and tells your future employers (hopefully) why you're the best person for the role. Standing out from the pack means knowing how to compile a winning application.

READ THE ADVERTISEMENT

Obvious, but often overlooked. Carefully studying the job ad will tell you exactly what employers are looking for in a prospective candidate. Make a list of all the qualities they're expecting you to demonstrate, and then tick them off as you write your application. If you have experience with a particular kind of software, and this is a key element of the job, it makes sense to pay it special attention. On the other hand, if something is not mentioned in the advertisement, it's probably best left out. Some might find your love of croquet simply fascinating, but it's unlikely to get you over the line for an IT job.

BE SPECIFIC

A job application is not the place to bang on about how much everyone loved you in your previous office, or how your jokes used to just kill at the water cooler. No-one cares. Instead, save room for the stuff that really matters. Keep in mind your prospective employers will probably end up sifting through dozens or even hundreds of vaguely similar applications, so get to the point quickly. Your application should be no longer than a couple of pages, unless specifically requested in the advertisement. Go for a brief introductory profile to tell them who you are, and then a chronological list of previous roles, with a brief explanation of what you did at each one. Rather than detailing every single task you did on a given workday, be specific about what you achieved and how it makes you a good candidate for the role – accomplishments like raising sales by 150 per cent, or cutting costs by 20 per cent. These are the kinds of concrete facts that stand out to employers more than describing yourself in vague clichés, like being 'enthusiastic' or a 'team player'.

DON'T LIE

While it's tempting to pretend you've already got a couple of Nobel Prizes under your belt, it's likely to do your job prospects more harm than good. Managers tend to follow-up on claims you make in your application – particularly if they're important components of the job. If you say you have skills you actually don't, it's going to become hard to conceal if you end up in the role. Being caught out also means that your application will be thrown out, and you'll be all but blacklisted from future job offerings. Avoid outright lies, but don't be afraid to emphasise anything that might help your prospects, and shift the focus from those that won't. Other key mistakes include spelling errors – especially the name of the company you're applying to – and grammatical slip-ups. Read over your application carefully before you send it.

MAKE IT PRESENTABLE

Compiling all your relevant information and experience is one thing, but the next step is to make sure it's easy to read and stands out from the other applications. Large blocks of text can be off-putting and easy to gloss over, so opt for key information in bullet points, with short explanatory paragraphs. Make headings bold, but don't include too many different colours or fonts, which can make it look like a high school project. Finally, make your name and contact details stand out, somewhere at the top of the page.

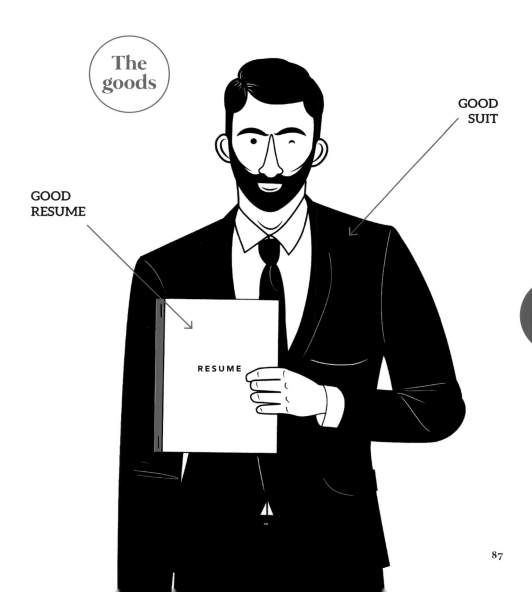

The goods

GOOD SUIT

GOOD RESUME

RESUME

FIVE

THE AVERAGE AMERICAN WORKER WILL HAVE AROUND 15—20 JOBS OVER THE COURSE OF THEIR WORKING LIFE.

THE INTERVIEW

They liked your application, and now they actually want to meet you in person. Hard to believe. But before you put the Champagne on ice, it's time to do a little work to make sure they fall in love with you. While few people like talking about how brilliant they are, this isn't the time to be shy. Instead, it's your opportunity to tell employers why you're the best one for the job, and show them a bit of your personality while you're at it. But you only get one chance at a first impression, so pay attention.

PREPARATION

One of the key reasons people come unstuck during job interviews is that they simply haven't done their homework. Find out as much as you can about the company and re-read the job advertisement to get an idea of the questions they are likely to ask. Other than that, it goes without saying that you want to look the part on the day. A nice suit and tie is usually the best option, and remember that it's better to be overdressed than under. You don't want to be late, either, so make sure you know the address, and how to get there ahead of time.

KEY QUESTIONS

While you can't know exactly what they're going to ask you, you don't have to be Nostradamus to guess the kinds of information they'll probably want to know. Most employers rely on the same old chestnuts in job interviews – here are a few you can expect, and how to handle them:

'Can you tell us a bit about yourself?'
This might seem like a chance to fill them in on that time you went to Europe after high school, but you want to keep it pretty business focused. Talk about where you studied and any notable achievements, as well

as how long you've been in the field, and what you enjoy about it. Feel free to mention any relevant hobbies, if they show your passion for the job.

'What attracted you to the position?'
This is the time to use all that research you've already done on the company, and explain why you're best suited to it. You can talk about your previous experience, and how well it fits with what the company does.

'What are your strengths and weaknesses?'
Strengths are fairly easy to talk about. But keep in mind you want to mention specific pursuits you're good at and then demonstrate why – it could be that you know you have strong leaderships skills because your team's sales increased by 20 per cent at your previous role. Weaknesses are trickier. The idea is to mention something you haven't done so well in the past, and then explain the steps you've taken to improve in that area.

It could be a training course you've taken, or an instance where you sought advice from your superiors.

'Do you have any questions?'
'No' is the wrong answer. Preparing questions ahead of time makes you seem enthusiastic and genuinely curious about the role. You might want to ask them what they see as the best feature about working at the company, what an average day tends to be like, or who they think the ideal candidate for the role is. Probably steer clear of quizzing them on why the last person left, or where the nearest pub is.

FOLLOWING UP
After the interview, send your potential employers a quick follow-up email to thank them for their time. Even if you don't end up landing the job, it's a chance for you to stay in their minds, in case any other opportunities do come up.

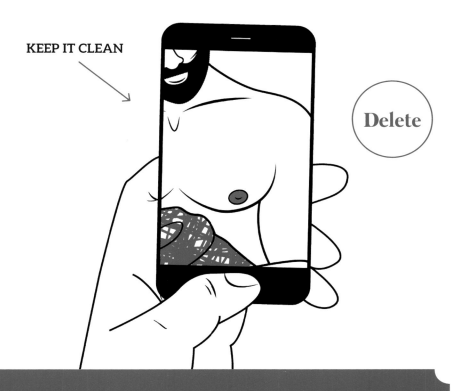

KEEP IT CLEAN

Delete

SOCIAL MEDIA

Unless you're applying for a position at an Amish commune, your employers will almost certainly have Googled you. Take a look through your social media accounts and eliminate anything immediately incriminating – drunken photographs, your appreciation of Nickelback's early years, etc. – though it's best to ensure any online accounts are set to private anyway.

ASKING FOR A PAY RISE

Pretty much everyone would like to be earning more than they are, but asking for a higher pay packet can be stressful or awkward – or both. Still, learning how to negotiate is a crucial part of climbing the corporate ladder. After all, it's about being rewarded for the hard work you've been putting into your career – and if you never ask, you'll always be left wondering what could have been. Here's how to approach the situation with the best chance of coming out on top.

TIME YOUR APPROACH

One of the most important aspects of negotiating a raise is to choose the right time to strike. If the company's profits are in freefall and the stock price is in the toilet, maybe it's not the ideal moment to waltz into your boss's office and demand more money. Instead, choose times when the business is doing well, or at least seems to be, especially if you've played a major part in bringing about some of that good fortune. While many presume raising the issue during their yearly evaluation is the best time, that's not always the case, as pay rises have often been decided well in advance.

BE CONVINCING

Know what you want, justify why you deserve it and anticipate the kinds of questions you might be asked to explain your request. If the best reason you can come up with is that you've heard Bora Bora is nice this time of year, the meeting will probably head south pretty quickly. Explain what you've brought to the business, and why you think you've exceeded any relevant performance indicators. Remember that pretty much everyone does tasks that go slightly above and beyond the strict definition of their job title, so focus on milestones in your professional development – taking on leadership roles, or making decisions that have directly benefited the company.

DON'T GET CARRIED AWAY

You want your offer to come across as serious. Asking for a huge pay rise out of the blue is not only likely to be met with a resounding no, but it's also going to make you seem greedy, possibly out of your mind, and like a poor candidate for any future pay rise opportunities. Standard pay rises tend to be between 1 and 5 per cent per year, so going much beyond that might be pushing your luck. Also, keep in mind this is a negotiation, so come in with a realistic offer and be prepared to listen to their counter argument. If it is a firm 'no' and there's no wriggle room, ask if they'd be willing to review the decision in a few months' time.

RESIGNING

Everyone's dreamed of going out in a blaze of glory. But as fun as it sounds, truth is, there's little to be gained from smashing your computer, telling your boss to kindly go screw themselves, and then stealing all the Post-It notes on your way out.

DON'T BURN YOUR BRIDGES

No matter how much of a colossal dick your boss is, it's handy for your work history to reflect ongoing relationships with previous employers because it suggests you're probably not a complete psychopath. Plus, staying in touch with them means they can keep you posted on better job opportunities, if they come up in the future.

Instead of going out with a bang, think of resigning as a natural part of your work life, especially given that the days of staying with the same company for decades on end are largely over. If you've got a better offer or you've just been in one place for too long, resigning with dignity is the smart way to go. Changing jobs is still the best way to increase your salary, and it's also a good way of finding out exactly how much you're worth.

READ YOUR CONTRACT

Before you kick off proceedings, make sure you know exactly how much notice you need to give and any other requirements of leaving. Also, get a new job. There aren't many reasons to leave one position unless you have another one to go to. Not only does it give you the safety of an actual income (handy!), it also lets you know where you stand if your current company comes back with another offer.

Speaking of, ask yourself what it would take to stay – whether it's a tasty pay rise, or a more senior role.

You should be able to answer that question before you go in, otherwise you may be put on the back foot, or miss a valuable opportunity for career advancement that doesn't involve leaving the company you're already with. Boring bureaucratic or monetary reasons, like having to train a new person, or paying out any holidays that are still owed, might prompt your company to try and keep you. Use them in your favour and be prepared for your manager to come back to you with a bid to encourage you to stay.

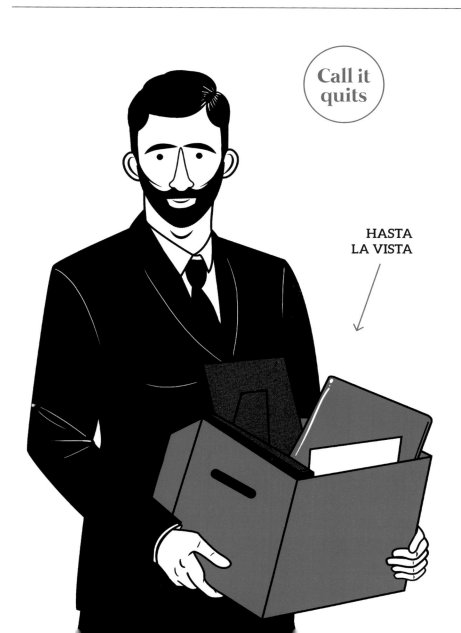

95

OFFICE POLITICS

While many workplaces may seem like bland cubicle farms, don't let that fool you. They're hotbeds of careful negotiation, minefields of diplomacy. It might seem like the sensible option is to stay out of any office politics altogether, but that's easier said than done. If you're new to a workplace, the best move is to fly under the radar for at least the first couple of weeks. Monitor those around you, listen to what they have to say and try not to offer too many of your own opinions until you know how to handle people. Best not to mention your previous job, if you can help it – and particularly not the way you used to handle tasks there. Believe it or not, people don't like to be told they're doing their job the wrong way by someone they've literally just met. Instead, make a list of potential changes you have in mind, and tackle them gradually, once you've settled in. Take some time to work out who's who around the office, and the best way to approach them. Here are a few characters to look out for:

THE GOSSIP

If you've heard the rumour about Becky having her fingers in the petty cash again, chances are it's arrived courtesy of this loud mouth. It doesn't actually matter if what they say is true (it's probably not) because once office gossip flares up, it's almost impossible to extinguish. Keep them onside as a valuable source, but don't get caught spreading their information.

THE CREDIT THIEF

You work overtime to get a project done on deadline, only to realise people thought it was a joint effort. These are the people who sneakily get the credit for others' work, but are nowhere to be seen when it all goes wrong. You need to look out for yourself by making sure people know exactly what you're working on, so they'll notice when someone sidles in

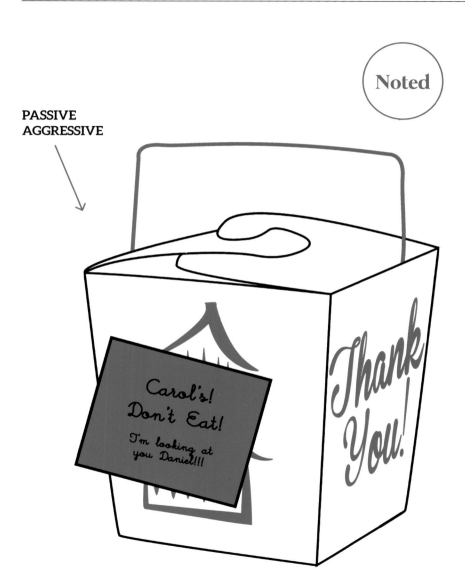

and tries to take the glory from under your nose.

THE TROUBLEMAKER

Forever trying to start office feuds, they're like The Gossip, but more nefarious. They'll try to get you to make negative comments about your colleagues, before telling everyone you're the one causing trouble. If you find yourself being quizzed about what you think of your colleagues, stick to one-word answers and don't let them bait you into dishing dirt on others.

THE VETERAN

They've been with the same company since the dawn of time, and they don't handle change well. Or at all. Approach with caution, but don't get them off side because they're not going anywhere. You might need them one day.

THE SYCOPHANT

Watch your mouth – and your back. Anything you say will almost certainly get back to the top brass. Always stick to office protocol, and don't complain about your job or co-workers because they'll be all too happy to make themselves look good by bringing you down. They've probably got your boss's ear, so don't be afraid to keep them on side – your good work might be noted further up the line.

THE MICROMANAGER

Even though their own ascent of the corporate ladder has been slower than they'd hoped, that hasn't stopped this frustrated middle-manager from pretending to be in charge and controlling every last detail of your day. They're the one perching over your shoulder to watch you write emails; drowning you in meaningless paperwork; or chastising you for turning up to work a full 37 seconds after 9 am. Don't complain. Instead, happily complete their menial tasks, safe in the knowledge that they're not going anywhere fast. One day you'll be their boss and you can return the favour.

'PLEASURE IN THE JOB PUTS PERFECTION IN THE WORK.' — ARISTOTLE

CHAPTER SIX
LEISURE

You know what they say about all work and no play. This chapter will have you covered on pastimes, from travel and social media to getting in shape and letting your hair down.

Now that you've done all the hard work, equipping yourself with the skills to live life to its fullest, it's time to relax. But it's not all fun. This chapter will cover everything from how to pick your ultimate holiday destination and pack your suitcase (the right way), navigate the online minefield that is social media, have some fun, and get back in shape – without going overboard.

TRAVEL

Experiencing the world is one of life's great luxuries. You get to soak up exotic cultures, see new sights, and experience the pure joy that is airport security screening. These few tips will give you the smarts you need to pack your suitcase, plan your ultimate holiday destination and score an upgrade.

BUCKET LIST

Let's say money was no object. Where would you visit? Even though your chances of becoming a millionaire overnight are slim, that doesn't mean you shouldn't start planning your ideal travel location. After all, cheap flights often come up at short notice. Whether you're a city dweller or enjoy nothing more than a spot of camping, turn the page for a simple guide that will help you choose the destination of your dreams, with 100 per cent accuracy*.

*OK, not really.

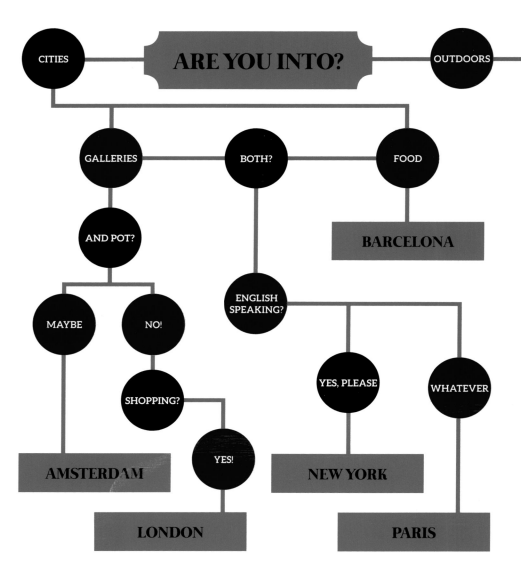

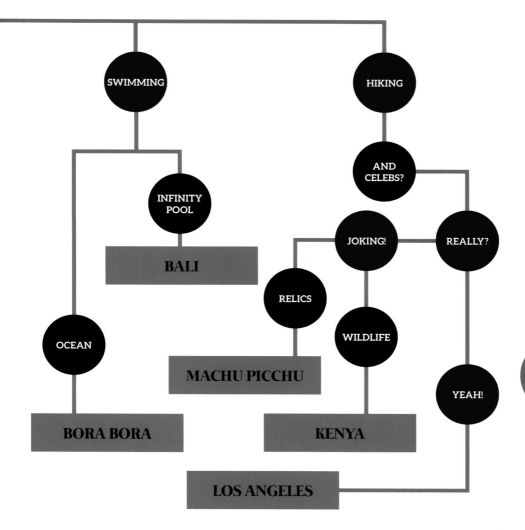

SWIMMING

HIKING

INFINITY POOL

AND CELEBS?

BALI

JOKING!

REALLY?

RELICS

OCEAN

WILDLIFE

MACHU PICCHU

YEAH!

BORA BORA

KENYA

LOS ANGELES

SIX

PACKING A SUITCASE

Everyone has a different technique, and while there might not be a consensus on how to do it, there are a few basic rules you should keep in mind next time you're due to head off on holiday. You lucky bastard.

PLAN AHEAD

First, find out if you require a visa, and get your paperwork approved well ahead of time to avoid any bureaucratic nightmares. Check the weather forecast of your destination for all the days you will be there – especially during the evenings. This might seem obvious but people often assume a place that tends to be warm will always be like that. Make a list of all the stuff you will need to take, including toiletries, under-wear, jackets, jumpers, trousers and electronics – including power adapters for different countries. Find out what your airline allows you to check-in (and what it doesn't) so you don't have any surprises at the airport. Items like hair dryers are awkward to pack and are usually available at most hotels, so avoid taking one if you can. Don't forget to weigh your luggage to avoid any nasty baggage fees at the airport.

ROLLING V FOLDING

Put some plastic bags in any shoes you're taking, and then fill with rolled-up socks and underwear. Put any nice shoes in dust bags, and then place at the bottom of your suitcase. Rolling clothes will make them more likely to crease, but will save you a lot of room. Folding your clothes will use more space, but will stop them creasing as much. Often, it's better to use a combination of the two techniques: rolling for items like T-shirts and jeans, which can often survive a few creases, and then folding for dress shirts and trousers.

'EVERY NOW AND THEN GO AWAY, HAVE A LITTLE RELAXATION, FOR WHEN YOU COME BACK TO YOUR WORK YOUR JUDGMENT WILL BE SURER.' — LEONARDO DA VINCI

SIX

CARRY ON

If you're heading overseas, you'll need to take your passport. Don't forget that. If your airline allows, a garment bag is a handy way to sneak in any items that didn't fit in your carry-on, or that need extra protection.

If you're travelling long-haul, try to bring a smaller toiletries bag in your hand luggage, with a deodorant, moisturiser and maybe a small cologne. Just be sure to check your airline's liquid limits beforehand.

You might also want to bring a change of clothes or underwear. Keep your passport on you at all times, and consider bringing a phone or laptop charger, and pens for any mid-transit paperwork. You can never have too many pens.

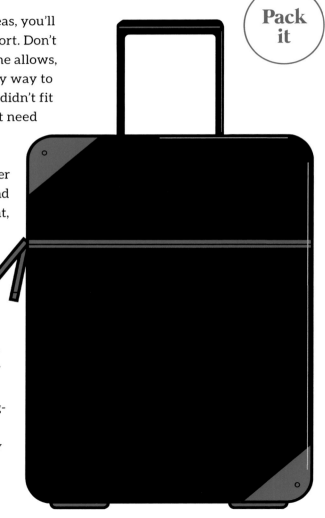

Pack it

GETTING
AN UPGRADE

The Holy Grail of airline travel. Everyone dreams of getting the nod to turn left instead of right as they walk on the plane. The reality is, it's probably not going to happen, but here are a few tips that might put the odds in your favour:

- Join the airline's frequent flyer program. They're likely to reward loyal customers.
- Travel alone. The chances of getting an upgrade are slim; the likelihood of getting two is non-existent.
- Dress the part. You're more likely to land a spot in first or business if you look like you belong there. That means maybe a casual blazer and jeans, rather than your usual tracksuit and sneakers (trainers) combination.
- Avoid business routes. People travelling for work often have a mountain of loyalty points, and will be an airline's first pick if an upgrade comes up. Holiday destinations are less likely to be swamped by business passengers, so you have a better chance of being chosen.
- Be nice. And get to the check-in counter early.
- Just ask. Politely enquire if there is any chance of an upgrade, remembering that there's no harm in asking.

SIX

SOCIAL MEDIA

Try as you might, it's all but impossible to avoid social media. While you might never be on the level of the Taylor Swifts and various Kardashians of the world, it pays to throw your hat in the ring. Not only does it help build a profile, which can help you professionally, but it's also a handy way to stay informed and build networks. Here are just a few tips to keep in mind to make sure you navigate the social media world and come out on top.

PRIVACY

Don't post anything on social media you wouldn't show your own mother. It's also worth setting your accounts to 'private', so only close friends can see what you post. This is about more than simply stopping people from seeing snaps of the poached eggs you had on the weekend; online security is a big deal, since people can easily glean information from your profile that can be used for potential identity theft. There's also all the other usual internet safety precautions to keep in mind: use bookmarks or the social network's web address, rather than email links; choose a complicated password that's not the same one you use for other accounts – especially email; and pick a username close to your actual name, to avoid people impersonating you.

COURTESY

Don't post anything about other people without their permission. This goes for the photos of them at that Christmas party where they drank all the champagne and ended up in a gutter. Hilarious, but poor form. When it comes to your own posts, ask yourself if the world really does need another shot of the poached eggs you had for brunch. Posting too often can be irritating, so be careful not to overshare.

You may feel the need to tell the world about absolutely everything going on in your life – but it might not appreciate an update on your ongoing haemorrhoid situation. Also, the online sphere is full of angry people hiding behind keyboards, so don't fight back if someone does send you a mean comment. Just delete it and move on.

OUTRAGE!

It's the internet, so everyone is angry, all the time. Being offended has become a worldwide hobby, with people keen to explain just how furious they are in 140 characters or less. Your jokes might seem hilarious when you tell them to your friends, but in the cold hard light of a computer screen, the humour might not come across quite as you intended. People are quick to take offence, and minor disagreements can turn into viral, public stonings very quickly. Don't let this dissuade you, but best to err on the side of caution.

NOT THE BOSS!

Nothing takes the fun out of social media quite like your boss following your account. It means ditching all the juicy stuff, as you're forced to upload posts about how much you enjoy working long hours. ('The stars looks so beautiful from my office window! #LoveMyJob.') You might even feel compelled to like all the photos of the incredibly lame holidays they take. If ignoring their follow request isn't an option, consider starting two accounts: one professional and one private. All the boring stuff is for your work account, while the Vegas trips and tequila shots go on the other. Just don't mix them up.

SIX

PARTY TIME

This is your chance to finally let your hair down. As long as you watch your manners (and don't hit the free bar too hard), you'll be able to have a great evening – without ruining everyone else's. Plus, play your cards right and with a bit of luck, the party invitations will keep coming well into the future. Now, let's get the party started.

THE INVITATION

If you've been formally invited to an event, an RSVP is not optional. The hosts are probably planning catering and drinks based on how many people will be attending, so simply turning up unannounced is not a good look. Also, don't bring anyone who hasn't been invited because not only will they throw the head-count out, but there could be a very good reason why their invitation was 'lost in the mail'. Be sure to indicate any dietary requirements if it's going to be a sit-down dinner, but don't be too picky – we're talking allergies or being vegetarian, rather than the fact you're not the biggest fan of tomatoes. Pay attention to any dress codes listed, but remember it's better to be overdressed than under.

THE ARRIVAL

Get there on time, which is to say slightly after the time on your invitation. If the event starts at 7 pm, arriving around 7.30 pm is the best option. Though if the invitation lists a finishing time, it's best to play it by ear – if it goes for just a couple of hours, get there closer to the listed start time; if it's due to kick on well into the early hours, you might want to push out your arrival another 30 minutes. Never get to an event before the starting time – it's not only rude, but will also probably be awkward, since you'll almost

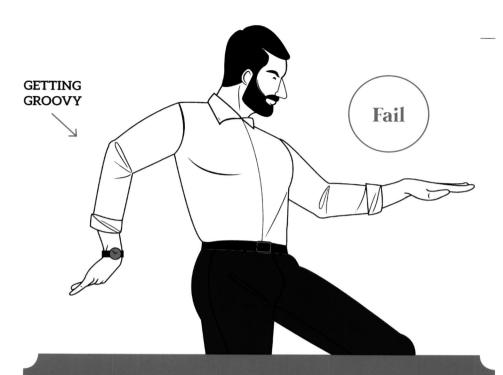

GETTING
GROOVY

Fail

DANCING

Most men can't dance. And that's not to say they're no Fred Astaire –
I mean they're not even in the ballpark. Rhythm might be something
you're born with, but here are a few mistakes to avoid:

Hands: Gun fingers are not the answer. Also, keep a strict below-the-
shoulders policy with your arms, to avoid humiliation or harming
others.
Face: Don't wink at other people. It's just weird.
Legs: Move with the hips, not the knees or feet.

SIX

certainly be stuck by yourself. Bringing a gift is a nice gesture, even if it's something small like a bottle of wine.

THE ARRIVAL

Greet the host when you arrive – though don't interrupt them if they're deep in conversation with another guest. Instead, try to catch their eye and allow them to come over to you. If you don't know many people, try to mingle with others, instead of hanging with the few people you do recognise.

THE CONVERSATION

The first step in meeting new people is remembering their name. Repeat it to yourself, or include it as a response when you're introduced to them: 'Nice to meet you, Janet.' Small talk doesn't have to be a chore. Before you get there, prepare a few topics that you're comfortable discussing in addition to what you do for a living, since people will probably ask that anyway. Things like travel or recent

exhibitions or concerts you've seen are classics. Make sure you give people something to work with, instead of sticking to single-word responses. Don't be afraid of pauses in conversation, but if things do get awkward, talking about the decor or music is a good fallback plan, as is asking how they know the hosts.

Don't feel bad about moving on if you get stuck with someone you'd rather not spend the evening chatting to. Just tell them you've spotted someone you should say hello to – failing that, heading to the bathroom is a good escape route.

THE EXIT

Don't linger too long. If the invitation lists a finishing time, aim to leave slightly beforehand, otherwise keep an eye on the room to see when other people make a move. If around half the party have left, things are probably winding down. After the event, send a thank-you note or some flowers to show your appreciation.

'I HAVE TO GO OUT EVERY NIGHT. IF I STAY HOME ONE NIGHT I START SPREADING RUMOURS TO MY DOGS.'
— ANDY WARHOL

SIX

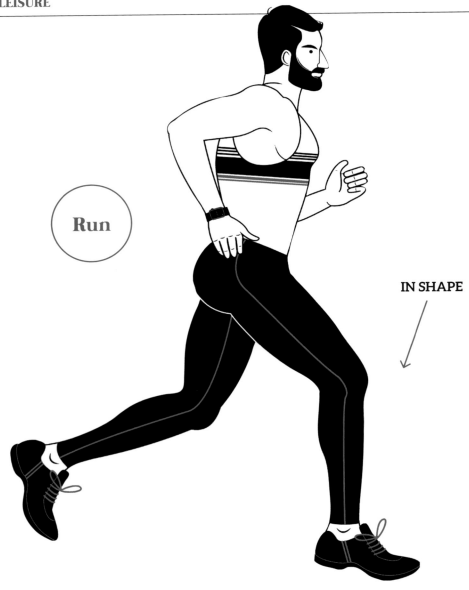

Run

IN SHAPE

HEALTHY LIVING

You're no spring chicken anymore. Your knees are shot, your back is sore and your joints pop like a series of tiny firecrackers every time you stand up. But getting yourself in shape before you grow old is not just a matter of looking your best. Eat well, exercise more, get enough shut-eye and cut down on the drinking, and your body will serve you well for years to come.

DIET

You can get away with eating whatever you want when you're younger, but it's only a matter of time before the pizza and beer start adding up. Being conscious of what you put in your body is not just about watching your weight, but also about your general health and wellbeing. Avoid eating too many processed foods, and replace saturated fat with good fats and oils found in foods like salmon, avocado and nuts. Instead of dieting, treat yourself to the things you really love but try to limit them to a certain number of times a week – instead of avoiding and then binging on them when you give in. Try to make fresh vegetables and cereals like whole grains the bulk of your diet, followed by lean meats and fish, then fruit and dairy.

EXERCISE

Being active is not simply about losing weight – though it helps – but also about the health benefits you gain from getting off the couch. Getting into exercise is a marathon, not a sprint – though maybe not an actual marathon, if you haven't been to the gym in a while. Take it gradually – starting at even 15 minutes a day, and then setting yourself achievable goals. If you find it hard to get motivated, get a friend on board to help keep you company, and to give you another reason to avoid hitting the snooze

SIX

THE GLOBAL HEALTH AND WELLNESS INDUSTRY IS ESTIMATED TO BE WORTH US$1 TRILLION.

button. It might also help to get an activity monitor or fitness tracking bracelet, which will keep track of your progress and show you your results in real time.

SLEEP

Seven hours a night is best practice. But life often gets in the way. If you do have trouble sleeping, avoid any screen activity in the hour before bedtime and try not to use your bed for anything other than sleeping and sex. Working on your laptop in bed might be comfy, but you don't want your mind to associate the bedroom with work when you're trying to nod off.

BOOZE

It probably sounds a bit rich coming from someone who just told you how to make five different cocktails – hold on, while I finish my martini ... there – but the truth is, alcohol is like anything: fine in moderation, but can become an issue if it gets out of hand. Try to keep a lid on the number of seriously boozy nights you have, rather than going through periods of binging and abstinence. Guidelines vary, but some classify heavy drinking as more than 14 units of alcohol a week, or more than four in one day. Keep in mind a bottle of beer contains around one standard unit of alcohol, and a glass of wine has at least 1.4.

RELAX

Everyone goes through difficult periods, but chronic stress can have very real effects on your wellbeing, from headaches and anxiety to high blood pressure and heart disease. Try to make time every day to rest your mind – whether it's going for a run, getting a massage, listening to music or meditating. If the problem is one that is ongoing, it's best to talk to a professional.

SIX

MAN
SKILLS

CHOPPING WOOD

Real men chop wood! Or something like that. If you feel like impressing others with your axe technique, here are a few pointers:

1. Get some gloves, decent work shoes and maybe some safety glasses (depending on your technique).
2. Find a solid chopping block to place your wood on. You want something solid and flat, but don't use anything without give, like concrete, or you'll damage your axe.
3. Position the wood vertically on top, then face it with your legs shoulder-width apart.
4. When gripping the axe, place your dominant hand above your non-dominant hand.
5. Bring your axe up over your dominant shoulder, and aim at any cracks in the wood.
6. Swing downwards and split the log. Repeat as necessary.
7. Congratulations! You've got firewood.

STARTING A FIRE

It's a skill we've been mastering for hundreds of thousands of years. So you'd think we'd have nailed it by now. Still, if you need a little help ...

1. Get an ignition source (a lighter or matches are the most obvious); some tinder (dry leaves, bark or paper); some kindling (small dry twigs); and some dry logs.
2. Clear a circular area about 1.2 m (4 ft) in diameter, and surround with logs or rocks to prevent the fire from spreading.
3. Pile kindling loosely in the middle, close enough to ignite but with enough room for air to circulate.
4. Place your tinder on the kindling and set alight.
5. Slowly add more kindling, while blowing gently on the small fire.
6. Add some logs, starting with small pieces, piled lengthways over the flames.
7. Build a 'teepee' with some extra logs by leaning the pieces of wood against one another.
8. Add more firewood, as required.

SEWING A BUTTON

Losing a button doesn't have to mean a trip to the tailor. Fixing it yourself is a much easier, cheaper option, and it will take just a few seconds to master.

1. Take 30 cm (12 in) of thread, knot it at one end and thread the other end through the eye of a needle.
2. Make a stitch in the shirt around 3 mm (1/8 in) in length, then make another perpendicular to the first. It should look like a small cross.
3. Hold the button 3 mm (1/8 in) away from the shirt, and thread the needle through one hole, into the shirt and back down through the opposite hole. Repeat four times for each hole.
4. Wrap the thread horizontally around the short cord separating the button from the shirt. Do this two or three times to create a strong 'pillar' of thread.
5. If you have any leftover thread, simply snip if off and discard it.

CHANGING A TYRE

Getting a flat tyre is a pain, and waiting for someone else to deal with it can take hours. Practise a couple of times when you're not on the road.

1. Block the wheels on the opposite side of the car, to prevent the car from moving.
2. Remove the hubcap from the wheel you're replacing.
3. Use the wrench to loosen the nuts, but don't remove them entirely.
4. Assemble the jack, and place at a reinforced area of the car – often the spot below the door is best.
5. Slowly raise the car, completely unscrew the nuts, and remove the wheel using both hands.
6. Place the spare wheel on, and replace the nuts. Some spare tyres can only be driven safely at certain speeds, so check this before you get moving.
7. Lower the car, and fully tighten the nuts (you may need to stand on the wrench, in the horizontal position).
8. Reposition the hubcap, and don't forget to have the old tyre repaired or replaced.

MAKING A SPEECH

Many people think of public speaking as a fate worse than death, but talking to a group doesn't have to be painful, as long as you follow these few simple rules:

1. Identify your key message and stick to it rather than trying to cover too many bases and ending up rambling.
2. Know your audience and the topics, tone or sense of humour they'll respond to – and what they won't.
3. Edit carefully. There's nothing worse than someone overstaying their welcome at the microphone, so remember that less is always more.
4. Practise beforehand, and time yourself. It pays to read it aloud to someone else to get honest feedback on how it sounds.
5. Read it, then read it again. Try to recite as much of your speech as possible without looking at your notes.
6. Capture the audience's attention. Make eye contact and use humour, entertaining anecdotes or famous quotes to engage people and stop them nodding off.
7. Speak up. No-one wants to strain to hear a whisper.
8. Finish strongly. The basic structure of a speech should be: tell them what you're going to say; say it; tell them what you've said. Your conclusion should sum up any points you've made.

PARALLEL PARKING

Driving around looking for a front-in parking spot is a fool's game. Reversing into a space is made easy with these few easy steps:

1. Find a spot that's big enough for your car – with room to spare. Ideally, it should be around a third longer than your car length.
2. Turn on your indicator and pull in beside the car in front.
3. Stop.
4. Begin by slowly reversing and immediately turning the steering wheel all the way towards the curb. You should be looking backwards, over your shoulder as you do this.
5. Stop when you reach a 45 degree angle.
6. Return the steering wheel to the centre position and continue backing up.
7. Stop when your side mirror is level with the back of the car in front.
8. Turn the wheel all the way to the opposite side and reverse into the spot.
9. Straighten up as you finish pulling into the space and brake – before you hit the car behind you.
10. Drive forwards until you are mid-way between the two cars.
11. Get out, and join passers-by in admiring your impressive parking skills.

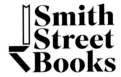

Published in 2016 by Smith Street Books
Melbourne | Australia
smithstreetbooks.com

ISBN: 978-1-925418-11-8

CIP data is available from the National Library of Australia.

Publisher: Paul McNally
Editor: Rachel Day
Design Manager: Joshua Beggs
Designer: Giuseppe Santamaria
Illustrator: Michael Sanderson

Printed & bound in China by C&C Offset Printing Co., Ltd.

Book 10
10 9 8 7 6 5 4 3 2 1